Top Curly Girl Products

Top Curly Girl Products

Copyright © 2019 by G.G Adshens.

Disclaimer and FTC Notice

The Methodology

Many curlies have gone on an endless product search for the perfect products for their curls, and ones that are curly girl method friendly at the same time in order to achieve the perfect curl, shine and moisture.

A global review was conducted looking at the following parameters:

- Global product usage with great reviews.
- Ease of access to product globally (international and local markets).
- Use of top rated natural ingredients that provide best benefits to curly hair including great curl definition.
- Curly girl method friendly products

Our review focused on two aspects that comprised, a deep research into the natural ingredients that go into the products that bring the ultimate benefit to curls of all hair types. This in combination with achieving superb curl definition as a result of using these selected natural ingredients.

The second aspect of the work was to review actual product use and reviews to see which formulations provided the best benefit to curls and their ease of access to the global curly community.

How to Use This Book

1.

Every curly is unique, and in the pursuit of finding what nature's best solution to your curls is, we have listed the main natural ingredients that have been guaranteed to work for various curl types. As you go through the natural ingredients we identified and their descriptions, have a try or review the ones you know you know your curls love.

This helps advise and help you narrow down on the products selection that work best for you.

2.

Highlighted in *italics* under each of the products listed are the top referenced natural ingredients contained in the product for curlies. This helps you narrow down to what you think may be the best combination for your hair.

3.

We have listed the top products found in the review in the following order

- Clarify
- Condition

- Style
- Spritz
- Detangle

4.

Choose the best products for your curls for each of the curly hair grooming stages, or experiment what your curls best respond to.

5.

For those who will still have a limited access to the products listed in this book based on geography and jurisdiction use the natural ingredients set out in this book to select the best product in your area. Be sure to make sure the products are silicone free (for conditioners), sulfate free (for clarifiers and shampoos) and alcohol free (for gels) in your searches. But you can use the top curly friendly natural ingredients in this book as a guide in your selections.

Table of Contents

Top Natural Ingredients Description

Coconut Oil

Coconut oil is highly moisturising, and therefore a great natural conditioner. It is also a great tonic for a dry and itchy scalp, including having unique antiviral, antifungal and antibacterial properties. Above all it restores dry, brittle and damaged hair, together with restoring split ends. This is particularly complementary for curly hair to make it frizz free and provide a perfect sleeked down look to achieve a perfect curl.

Further, coconut oil helps with boosting hair growth and infusing nutrients into your curly hair follicles. This leads to thicker hair and length retention. Coconut oil protects hair from heat and styling impacts by strengthening hair strands, making hair more resilient. It also adds luster, softness and shine to curly hair.

Aloe Vera

Aloe vera is exceptionally rich in vitamins, essential amino acids, copper, zinc and fatty acids which are essential for curly hair. Aloe vera uniquely has a similar pH to curly hair and has up to 96% water content within which all these nutrients are embedded. The nutrients help with healthy hair maintenance and hair growth.

Aloe vera is a great conditioner and can also be used as a detangler. It strengthens curly hair follicles and infuses shine and smoothness. The amino acids make the hair super soft and enhance curl definition with one application. Most importantly aloe vera helps hair retain water and moisture more than many other natural sources.

Olive Oil

Olive oil is exceptional in reducing brittleness and making hair soft and eliminate frizz. It is rich in fatty acids which benefit the hair, containing monounsaturated essential fatty acids, palmitic acid, oleic acid, squalene and terpenes. These are emollients and have the effect of softening and smoothening curls.

Olive oil contains vitamin E, which fights free radical damage from sunlight and pollution. Olive oil helps reduce dandruff by softening flakes and reducing inflammation and itching. Olive oil is able to penetrate hair stands and thereby deeply nourish and condition the hair from within. This helps lock in moisture and ensure softness, strength and shine.

Antioxidants in olive oil reduce inflammation on scalp and hair follicles and help with hair growth. It also helps with repairing split ends of hair and can help with visible improved appearance and smoothness of hair, including strengthening of hair cutting down on hair loss. Overall olive oil supports hair manageability of all curl types and helps make it easier to style and maintain. Its particularly

helpful for colour treated hair, frizz, brittle
and damaged hair.

Lemon Balm

Lemon balm or *Melissa officinalis* comes from the mint family, making it relatively similar to peppermint. It is a natural curly hair ingredient which supports curlies with oily hair or excessive sebum. It plays a big role in acting as a mild astringent to remove oiliness from the hair and scalp.

Further the tannin in lemon balm helps relieve an irritated and damaged scalp and has a highly soothing effect. It contains caffeic acid, ferulic acid and flavonoids enabling it to have antioxidant effects on hair and scalp. It is also great for hair loss, cleansing the scalp and dealing with scalp irritations.

Shea Butter

Shea butter comes from shea nuts from West Africa. Shea butter is rich in Vitamin A, E,F, D, essential fatty acids which include palmitic acid, stearic acid and oleic acid which boost moisture in curls. This significantly reduces dryness and split ends while nourishing the hair. It softens even the driest and most brittle hair and curl textures, making curls look more succulent. Shea butter strengthens hair fibres, lubricates and softens cuticles and significantly reduces frizz.

Shea butter helps reduce scalp irritation and unclogging of pores. It is good for protecting against sun and heat damage as well as sea salt at the beach.

Curly hair can lose moisture quickly, by applying shea butter, moisture is sealed in making hair extremely soft. It decreases hair loss and breakage through stimulation of collagen production and strengthening of hair strands.

Passion fruit

Passion fruit is a rich antioxidant which is rich in Vitamin A, C, B2, B6 including copper and potassium. These are important nutrients that help and support oxygen and nutrient delivery to hair follicles for succulent, healthy curls.

Passion fruit helps with hair strength, through formation of collagen and protecting hair from breakage and weakness. Passion fruit also helps strengthen curls alleviating and protecting hair from split ends. It is great for hair loss reduction.

The antioxidant nature of passion fruit nourishes the scalp and keeps it healthy. It supports healthy roots thereby strengthening the hair for long and strong hair. The vitamins in passion fruit helps improve the curl texture and curl definition of hair.

Bamboo extract

Bamboo extract is derived from the leaves and stems of bamboo. Bamboo is a natural replacement for silicone, and contains natural elements making it great for curly hair. It boosts shine, giving a healthy glow of hair. This property also helps seal in moisture and help nutrients enter the hair shaft. Bamboo adds a great sheen and luster to curly hair and leaves the hair strand smooth and silky to the touch.

Bamboo extract is effective in promoting hair growth as it is rich in silica which aids in speeding up growing of hair. It is also great for strengthening and making hair thicker. This extract is also known to be good for the skin and scalp improving circulation, which in turn strengthens hair follicles and promote thicker hair and growth.

Bamboo extract is great for cleansing hair to remove product build up and dirt from curls. This leaves your curls looking luscious and fresh.

Soybean oil

Soybean oil is important for moisture retention. Soybean oil contains lipids that help the hair take in moisture, including taking up conditioner and hair treatments effectively. In order to achieve a well defined curl structure moisture is required. Soybean oil aids in increasing moisture intake and retention in the hair, making it a great curly natural ingredient.

Soybean also increases shine and leads to longer lasting curl definition and structure. It is very nourishing due to its rich vitamin and nutrient content. The more nourished your curls are the softer the hair, and easier to manage with reduced frizz.

With regular of soybean oil use, curls are strengthened through its protein content.

Hops

Hops extract is extremely helpful for the treatment of the scalp and elimination of dandruff. The oils and vitamins found in hops help to open pores of the scalp to reduce loss of hair. The oils also help repair scalp and ensure healthy hair follicles.

When hops extract is used in combination with other curly friendly natural oils such as olive oil, coconut oil, the curls have improved shine and strength. Combination of hops and other natural or essential oils improves the appearance, shine and health of curls.

Sweet Almond Oil

Sweet almond oil is rich in omega fatty acids, Vitamin E and protein which improves the strength and shine of hair. It acts a sealant, hair protector and emollient which fills in hair cuticles and makes hair smooth to the touch. Prolonged use of sweet almond oil allows for a softer curl texture over time as the hair shaft is moisturised from the inside.

Almond oil helps with the repair of the hair shaft and strengthens your curls reducing breakage. This is effective for repair and management of split ends, by building resilience of the hair.

This oil is a great treatment for scalp conditions, including a dry scalp. It is full of powerful antioxidants that are beneficial to the skin and hair.

It also makes curls have a shine with a silky look.

Argan Oil

Argan oil is a deeply hydrating oil that promotes healthy hair. It improves the luster and texture of curls. Argan oil is rich in vitamin E, fatty acids and other antioxidants. Argan oil is well known for its anti-frizz ability and elimination of split ends. It is absorbed into curl structures with visible improved appearance and texture.

Argan oil helps with dry scalp conditions through its powerful antioxidant and anti-inflammatory ingredients to improve the scalp. It also soothes inflamed scalps and reduces dandruff.

It is effective in strengthening hair follicles and reduces hair loss with consistent use. Above all it is a great conditioner for curls, while moisturising the scalp and provides for exceptional for curl definition.

Rosemary

Rosemary is well known for its hair growth properties. It is known to have anti-inflammatory properties, while promoting nerve growth and circulation in the scalp, all which enhance hair growth. It also helps with dry and itchy scalp conditions.

Rosemary is good as a cleanser through its antibacterial properties which is a bonus when cleansing hair. It also improves curl shine for an improved glow of hair.

CLARIFY TOP PRODUCTS

Shea Moisture Organic Coconut and Hibiscus Curl and Shine Shampoo

(Coconut juice, Shea butter, Coconut oil, Aloe vera)

Provides, anti-frizz, moisture and shine for well-defined and bouncy curls. The coconut and neem oils in this product help with moisture retention and helps define curls with good body. Overall hydrates, reduces breakage, smoothes curls and controls frizz providing a great shine.

Shea Moisture Organic Raw Shea Butter Moisture Retention Shampoo

(Shea butter, Argan oil, Aloe vera, Coconut oil)

A sulfate free shampoo that moisturises dry, brittle and damaged hair. It contains key natural ingredients including coconut oil, aloe vera, shea butter, sea kelp and argan oil. It helps smooth hair cuticles and seal them, leaving curls smooth and with good curl definition. This shampoo restores shine and helps with elasticity, while being a great moisturiser at the same time.

Shea Moisture Professional Clear Start Shampoo

(Shea butter)

Helps define and lengthen even the tightest curls. The natural lipids in this product help block humidity. This is a sulfate free formulation which is great for removing build up, residue, chlorine build up and hard water minerals. This is also a good frizz protection formulation, and leaves hair soft and curls looking their best.

Devacurl Low Poo Delight

(Lemon balm, Hops, Rosemary)

This is a sulfate free gentle cleanser that aids with frizz control and removes oiliness and residue from curls. It is a light formulation that cleans the scalp and hair, leaving hair with body and defined curls. Overall this product helps with providing hair with fullness, bounce and definition.

CONDITION TOP PRODUCTS

Tressemme Botanique Nourish and Replenish Conditioner

(Coconut oil, Aloe vera)

This is a very nourishing conditioner which leaves hair smooth and silky. It is made of the top natural ingredients coconut milk and aloe vera. It is great for frizz control and smoothness, leaving hair silky soft and very well moisturised. It is also great for replenishing your hair with moisture when it becomes drier.

Matrix Biolage Conditioning Balm

(Aloe vera, Passion fruit)

This is a greatly moisturising conditioner that helps control frizz and deeply moisturises each curl strand of all curl types. It optimises moisture balance and leaves hair refreshed and hydrated. This moisturising and nourishing property leaves curls well hydrated with good curl definition. It is good for renewing moisture in the hair and reducing dryness and frizz.

Devacurl One Condition Original

(Olive oil, Lemon balm, Hops, Rosemary)

A creamy conditioner that is infused with olive oil for super softness and well hydrated hair. It is well nourishing and leaves hair soft, frizz free and shiny. Works well on all curl types and leaves curls well defined. Locks in hydration for manageable and defined curls.

Shea Moisture Raw Shea Butter Restorative Conditioner

(Shea butter, Argan oil, Coconut oil)

This is a great detangling conditioner and moisturiser. It provides life to lifeless, damaged and brittle curls. Infused with shea butter, argan oil and coconut oil it deeply moisturises and repairs hair. Is formulated and designed for all curl types, and aids with improved curl definition.

STYLE TOP PRODUCTS

Ecostyler Olive Oil Styling Gel

(Olive Oil)

This alcohol free gel is infused with 100% olive oil. Olive oil infuses moisture in curls while nourishing the hair and scalp. Has a great hold, weightless and leaves hair with a good shine. Provides great frizz control.

Other product ranges of ecostyler styling gel great for curl definition and frizz control include Black Castor and Flaxseed Oil, Argan Oil and Coconut Oil ranges.

Biotera Styling Gel

(Bamboo, Shea butter, Coconut oil, Sweet almond, Soybean oil)

This is a light gel with bamboo extract that provides curl definition and control with no stickiness or flaking. Contains nettle that strengthens and adds luster to curls. Good for curls needing body and bounce. The formulation strengthens and moisturises dry brittle hair.

Fantasia IC Hair Polisher Styling Gel

(Aloe vera)

Styling gel that contains aloe vera and provides great curl definition. Smoothes curls for a very natural look, with volume and shine. Enriched with aloe, wheat protein and spark lite conditioners.

Cantu Shea Butter Moisturising Curl Activator Cream

(Coconut oil, Shea butter, Aloe vera, Sweet almond oil, Olive oil, Argan oil)

Formulated with pure shea butter, activates curls leaving hair well defined. Smoothes and enhances curl pattern leaving bouncy curls with shine, infused with moisture. Good product for a wash and go. Great for a moisture infusion.

Aussie Instant Freeze Sculpting Gel

(Aloe vera)

Maximum hold styling gel that provides sculpt and shine. Infused with aloe vera, jojoba oil and sea kelp. Provides great definition and hold to curls. Great for frizz control and hold styles.

SPRITZ TOP PRODUCTS

Tressemme Botanique Nourish and Replenish Leave In Hydrating Mist

(Coconut oil, Aloe vera)

Enriched with aloe vera and coconut oil, this hydrating mist detangles dry hair and refreshes curls with infusion of softness. This mist provides a boost of hydration without weighing curls down, and leaves hair with a light bounce and good shine. Lightly detangles leaving curls well nourished and moisturised.

Devacurl Mist-er Right Dream Curl Refresher

(Lemon balm, Hops, Rosemary)

A revitalising spritz that helps boost curl definition and body. Curls look succulent, fresh and shiny with this refresher. Infused with lavender oil, has a good refreshing scent and helps bring life back to curls. Refreshes scalp and hair daily and between washes.

Shea Moisture 100% Virgin Coconut Oil Leave In Treatment

(Coconut oil, Shea butter, Argan oil)

This leave in treatment and spritz is a good detangler and provides for smoothing of hair and leaving curls tangle free. Highly infused with coconut oil it provides softness and shine to hair and has great moisturising and nourishing properties. Helps seal open split ends to keep curls frizz free.

Coconut oil contains Vitamin E which is highly moisturising for curls, while its triglyceride component helps with moisture retention. This treatment is good for smoothing and softening hair.

DETANGLE TOP PRODUCTS

Shea Moisture Raw Shea Butter Extra Moisture Detangler

(Shea butter, Argan oil, Coconut oil)

Mineral and nutrient rich detangler to easily detangle curls in a smooth way. The detangler smoothes and seals hair cuticles making it easy to undo knots and clumped hair. Deeply moisturises curls to make them manageable with nourishment. The argan oil in this formulation helps enhance shine to curls while conditioning and renewing hair.

Devacurl Washday Wonder

(Lemon balm, Hops, Rosemary)

A great pre cleanse to detangle hair before washing and conditioning your curls. Provides good slip to detangle hair, while strengthening and reducing breakage. The sweet almond oil rich in omega fatty acids and vitamins helps moisturise curls and provide nourishment. It is very effective in detangling knotted and matted curls. Best used alongside the No Poo/ Low Poo Cleanser and One Condition Original Conditioner in the Devacurl range.

Devacurl No Comb Detangling Spray

(Lemon balm, Hops, Rosemary)

This spray is a great water base product for detangling that is sprayed on the hair. The leave in spray untangles curls easily and is good for smoothing and frizz free curls. Adds shine to dull hair. Leaves curls smooth and well defined.

61370839R10018

Made in the USA
Middletown, DE
19 August 2019